HEART-HEALTHY SLOW COOKER RECIPE COOKBOOK

Delicious Recipes for a Healthy and Balanced Heart-Healthy Lifestyle

Contents

Overview of Cardiovascular Disease

The heart is an organ that is part of the circulatory system and is responsible for pumping blood throughout the body. It is composed of cardiac muscle, which is responsible for contracting and relaxing to pump the blood. The heart is made up of four chambers: the right and left atria and the right and left ventricles. The right side pumps deoxygenated blood to the lungs to be oxygenated, while the left side of the heart pumps oxygenated blood to the rest of the body.

Cardiovascular disease, also known as heart disease, is a group of conditions that affect the heart, blood vessels, and blood circulation. These diseases can lead to serious health problems such as heart attack, stroke, and heart failure. Common risk factors for heart disease include high blood pressure, high cholesterol, smoking, obesity, diabetes, and lack of physical activity.

A heart healthy diet is a diet that is rich in fruits, vegetables, low-fat dairy, whole grains, fish, nuts, and legumes and is low in unhealthy fats and sodium. Eating a heart healthy diet can help reduce the risk of developing cardiovascular disease. It can also help manage existing heart disease. Some of the benefits of a heart healthy diet include lower blood pressure, lower cholesterol, and improved heart health.

Eating a heart healthy diet is an important part of preventing and managing cardiovascular disease. It is important to focus on eating a variety of nutritious foods and limiting unhealthy fats and sodium. Eating a diet rich in fruits, vegetables, low-fat dairy, whole grains, fish, nuts, and legumes can help reduce the risk of developing cardiovascular disease and improve overall heart health.

Cardiovascular disease (CVD) is a leading cause of death and disability in the United States and worldwide. It is a term used to describe conditions affecting the heart, including coronary heart disease, stroke, and hypertension. CVD is a complex condition with multiple risk factors, including lifestyle choices, genetics, and age.

The anatomy and physiology of the heart play a major role in the development and progression of CVD. The heart is composed of four chambers, two atria and two ventricles, that contain blood. The heart's muscular walls contract and relax to pump blood throughout the body. The cardiac cycle is the series of events that occurs when the heart beats. The coronary arteries supply the heart with oxygen-rich blood.

CVD is a preventable condition. It is caused by a combination of lifestyle choices and risk factors, including genetics, age, and race. Smoking, physical inactivity, poor diet, and excessive alcohol consumption can increase the risk for CVD. High cholesterol and hypertension are also associated with an increased risk for CVD.

Fortunately, CVD can be prevented through lifestyle changes. Regular physical activity, stress management, and a heart healthy diet can reduce the risk for CVD. Exercise can help maintain a healthy weight, reduce stress, and improve overall health. Stress management is also important for reducing the risk for CVD.

A heart healthy diet is an important part of CVD prevention. A heart healthy diet is rich in fruits and vegetables, low-fat dairy, whole grains, fish, nuts, legumes, and healthy fats. It is also important to limit unhealthy fats and sodium.

In conclusion, CVD is a major cause of death and disability in the United States and worldwide. Its development and progression are influenced by the anatomy and physiology of the heart. CVD is a preventable condition with multiple risk factors, including lifestyle choices, genetics, and age. Exercise, stress management, and a heart healthy diet can reduce the risk for CVD. By following a heart healthy diet, people can reduce their risk for CVD and improve their overall health.

Risk Factors and Types of Cardiovascular Disease

Cardiovascular disease is a broad term used to describe conditions that affect the heart and blood vessels. It is a leading cause of death in the United States, and the risk factors for developing these diseases are numerous. This article will provide an overview of the various types of cardiovascular disease, as well as the risk factors associated with each.

Risk Factors

The most common risk factors associated with cardiovascular disease are smoking, high blood pressure, high cholesterol, obesity, physical inactivity, diabetes, and unhealthy eating habits. Other risk factors include age, gender, family history, and certain medications. It is important to note that some of these risk factors can be modified or eliminated altogether with lifestyle changes, such as quitting smoking and increasing physical activity.

Types of Cardiovascular Disease

There are several different types of cardiovascular disease, all of which can have serious health implications. The most common types of cardiovascular disease include coronary artery disease, congestive heart failure, stroke, and peripheral artery disease.

Coronary artery disease occurs when the arteries that supply blood to the heart become blocked or narrowed. This can lead to chest pain and an increased risk for a heart attack.

Congestive heart failure occurs when the heart is unable to pump enough blood to meet the body's needs. This can lead to shortness of breath, fatigue, and swelling in the legs and feet.

Stroke is a medical emergency that occurs when a blood vessel in the brain is blocked or bursts. This can lead to permanent disability or even death.

Peripheral artery disease occurs when the blood vessels in the legs become narrowed or blocked. This can lead to pain, numbness, and difficulty walking.

It is important to note that all of these conditions can have serious health implications, and it is important to take steps to reduce your risk of developing cardiovascular disease. This includes eating a healthy diet, getting regular exercise, quitting smoking, and controlling risk factors such as high cholesterol and high blood pressure.

In conclusion, cardiovascular disease is a serious health condition that affects millions of people each year. Knowing the risk factors and types of cardiovascular disease can help you take steps to reduce your risk and lead a healthier life.

What Do We Mean By Heart-Healthy?

A fair question is what we really mean by heart-healthy and how these recipes fit that description better than the ones in other slow cooker books. It seems like there is a lot of discussion and some controversy about what really is heart-healthy. But there are a couple of key concepts that I have come to believe in over the years that most mainstream medical people agree with as well.

They are as follows:

- Reduced sodium

- Reduced saturated fats and trans fats

- Less dietary cholesterol

- Higher fiber

Let's look at each of these in turn and see why these recipes adhere to these concepts.

Reduced Sodium

As many of you who are familiar with my other books or my website may know, reducing sodium was the first goal of my heart-healthy cooking journey. As a starting point, consider the following facts:

- The United States Food and Drug Administration recommends 2,300 milligrams (mg) of sodium daily for healthy adults.

- The US Department of Agriculture recommends that individuals with hypertension, African Americans, and adults 50 and older should consume no more than 1,500 mg of sodium per day.

- The United Kingdom Recommended Nutritional Intake (RNI) is 1,600 mg daily.

- The National Research Council of the National Academy of Sciences recommends 1,100 to 1,500 mg daily for adults.

- Studies have shown that many people in the United States and Canada routinely consume 2 to 3 times that amount.

Given these figures, it's pretty safe to say that many of us consume more sodium than is good for us. If you already have a history of heart disease or have a family history of it, it's even worse. I know I sound a bit like a zealot in this, but I can honestly say that I felt much better when I first started my lowsodium diet over 10 years ago. And I'm probably in a better position now medically than I was then. All I can say is that it's worked for me and for lots of other people I've talked to.

Reduced Saturated Fats and Trans Fats

These have been shown by a number of studies to be major contributors to high cholesterol. In general, saturated fats are fats that are solid at room temperature. There are several sources of saturated fats. The most common ones are the following:

•   Red meats—Beef, pork, and lamb contribute a significant amount of saturated fat to our diets. Many experts recommend reducing the amount of red meat we eat. If you find that difficult, and I admit that I do, the slow cooker can help by allowing you to use leaner cuts of meat.

• Poultry skin—Any slow cooker recipe you look at recommends removing the skin from poultry, thus problem solved.

• Whole fat dairy products—By using other items like cream soups and fat- free evaporated milk in our slow cooker recipes, you won't even notice that you aren't using whole milk or cream for that chowder.

• Tropical oils—We use only healthier oils like olive and canola and don't even miss things like palm and coconut oil.

Trans fats are also called trans-fatty acids. They are produced by adding hydrogen to vegetable oil through a process called hydrogenation. This makes the fat more solid and less likely to spoil. Research has clearly linked trans fats to a number of health problems. The most common sources are margarine and other solid shortenings. In general, I never use them.

Less Dietary Cholesterol

Although there has been some disagreement about how significant the role of eating foods high in cholesterol is in increasing your blood cholesterol, most experts still recommend reducing it. Common sources of dietary cholesterol are the following:

• Egg yolks—I almost never use whole eggs, preferring to use an egg substitute like Egg Beaters that is made from egg whites. I can't tell the difference.

- Organ meats—This is good news for everyone who hates liver. (I happen to like it, but I only eat it once every couple of months.)

- Shellfish—This is another thing I like but try to limit.

Higher Fiber

There have been a number of studies showing the benefits of increasing our fiber intake, not only for heart health, but for many other areas of the body as well. A few key findings are as follows:

- A study published in the May 11, 2000 issue of The New England Journal of Medicine reported that diabetic patients who maintained a very high-fiber daily diet lowered their glucose levels by 10 percent.

- A 1976 study by the Veterans Administration Medical Center in Lexington, Kentucky, showed that fiber is useful in treating diabetes, high blood pressure, and obesity and in reducing cholesterol levels.

- Two studies published in The Lancet showed that people with high fiber diets suffered from fewer incidents of colon polyps and colon cancer.

So there are a lot of good reasons to add more fiber to your diet, even if you aren't currently being treated for a medical condition that requires it.

In the next section I describe what we've done to bring these recipes in line with these guidelines.

How We Make Recipes Heart-Healthy

Most of the things we've done to make these recipes more heart-friendly involve simple substitutions and changes to the usual ingredients. Some may seem obvious, particularly to anyone who has read any of my other books. Some may be less so. The following are some of the key ones.

Eliminate the Salt

One question that may occur to some people looking over the recipes in this book is, "Why is there no salt in any of the ingredient lists?" That's a fair question and deserves an answer. As I said in the Introduction, I first got involved with heart-healthy cooking because my doctor put me on a lowsodium diet. It took some time and lots of experimentation, but I learned how to cook things that both taste good and are easy to prepare that are still low in sodium. Along the way, we literally threw away our salt shaker. There's one shaker full of light salt (half salt and half salt substitute) on the table. My wife uses that occasionally. Two of my children have given up salt completely, not because they need to for medical reasons, but because they are convinced like I am that it's the healthy thing to do. When I started creating recipes focused on other areas of heart health, going back to using salt wasn't even something I considered. In creating these recipes, I was not as strict about the amount of sodium as I usually am in my own diet. I didn't plan on people buying special sodium-free baking powder that is difficult to find except online. I didn't eliminate most cheeses except Swiss. But I also didn't add any salt. I think if you try the recipes, you'll find that they taste good without it. If you are tempted to add some salt because you think it's needed, I'd suggest that first you try the recipe and see whether you like it without the salt. And if you have trouble with the idea of giving up salt, you might check with your own doctor. I believe that most doctors will agree that in the interest of total health, you are better off without the salt.

Use Lower-Fat Meats and Dairy Products

I already talked about this, but the slow cooker makes it really easy because you can use lean meat, skinned poultry, and fat-free dairy products and no one will even notice.

Use Egg Substitute Instead of Whole Eggs

Again, this is a simple change, and one that won't be noticed. But it can significantly decrease the amount of cholesterol you eat.

Substitute Whole-Grain Products

I've discovered that I like whole-grain products better than the refined ones in most cases. You can use brown rice in place of white, whole-grain pasta, and other whole grains like barley in a number of these recipes. Many of these recipes make stews or other dishes with sauces that are even better over brown rice than white. Give it a try.

Use Healthier Fats

The only fats used in these recipes are healthier oils like olive and canola and unsalted butter. Yes, I know that butter has cholesterol that we are trying to hold down. But it is a lot easier to find than unsalted margarine. And considering the many health problems that may be linked to trans fats in our diet, I've made the personal decision that butter is probably healthier than margarine. Given the choice, I always try to go with the more natural product.

Substitute Healthier Ingredients

In some cases, this is as easy as reading the food labels and picking the healthier option. There are low-fat, lowsodium versions of many soups available. There are no-salt-added tomato products like sauce, paste, chopped and crushed tomatoes, and even ketchup. And they are all available at most large grocery stores. If you go to a store that specializes in organic and gourmet foods like Whole Foods or Trader Joe's, you'll find more options. Seek them out and you'll have more options yourself when looking at recipes.

But this is also where chapter 2 comes in. Many of the items in that chapter are not, in themselves, slow cooker recipes. But they are the building blocks that can allow you to easily create heart-healthy recipes in your slow cooker. For example, the first recipe is for a reduced-sodium soy sauce that contains only 33 mg of sodium per serving, about one-tenth what the lowest commercially available product contains. So now when a recipe calls for Y cup (60 ml) of soy sauce, you don't have to immediately discard it as something you are not allowed to have. Other recipes there include lowsodium chili and barbecue sauces, low-fat and lowsodium sausage, nosalt onion soup mix, seasoning blends and dressing mixes, and even a low- fat and lowsodium baking mix to use in place of Bisquick. I usually make these up in large quantities and store them in the refrigerator or freezer to have on hand. I realize that depending on where you live it may not be easy to find heart-healthy options on your grocer's shelves. So my answer is, "If you can't find it, make it."

Why the Slow Cooker Is Good for Heart-Healthy Cooking

Of course, as I said at the beginning of this introduction, there is nothing inherently healthy about slow cooker cooking. But there are a few features that you can take advantage of that make the slow cooker a friend in your quest to eat heart-healthy.

Perhaps the most readily noticeable thing is that it's easier to cook lower- fat recipes in the slow cooker. Not only do leaner cuts of meat cook well in the slow cooker, they actually cook better, ending up more tender and with more flavor than if you cook them by conventional means. Cooking lean meat quickly often toughens it, while boiling it breaks it down to the point where it has no flavor. Long, slow cooking makes it tender and keeps the flavor, the ideal situation. You'll find that the beef recipes in this book usually call for the lean cuts like round steak or roast, which are both lower in fat and cheaper. On the chicken side of the aisle, most recipes recommend that you remove the fat and skin before slow cooking. This also supports our desire to cut back on saturated fats since the skin is where most of the fat in poultry resides.

But perhaps the biggest advantage is one that is not so obvious. One of the most common things I hear from many people that prevents them from cooking heart-healthy meals is that is takes time. If you are serious about reducing your sodium eating less fat, increasing the amount of fiber in your diet, you will almost certainly have to cook more things from scratch. You just aren't going to find that kind of nutrition in the quick and easy prepackaged mixes and frozen dinners. However, the slow cooker can cut your preparation time, particularly in the evening when you are tired and don't feel like cooking. You can throw things in it in the morning, and when you get home, dinner is ready. Or if you want to make something like pasta sauce that benefits from long, slow cooking, the slow cooker can handle that unattended. And that is a real advantage that making things from scratch the conventional way does not offer.

Tips for Slow Cooker Success

The following tips will help to ensure that you are pleased with the result of your slow cooking. (Yes, I know that some of the recipes in this book don't follow all these rules.)

- Fill the slow cooker one-half to two-thirds full. If you fill it to the top, foods may not cook properly or will take longer to cook. If the level is lower, the foods may cook too quickly. If you cook for different numbers of people at different times, you may want to have several slow cookers of different sizes.

- Don't lift the lid, especially if you are cooking on the low setting. Each time you lift the lid, enough heat will escape that the cooking time should be extended by 20 to 30 minutes.

- For safe cooking, always thaw meat or poultry before putting it into a slow cooker. Frozen food takes too long to thaw and get to a safe cooking temperature.

- Foods cooked on the bottom of the slow cooker cook faster and will be more moist because they are immersed in the simmering liquid.

- Fresh root vegetables, such as potatoes, carrots, and onions should be placed in the bottom of the pot, under the meat, for faster cooking. They tend to cook more slowly than meat. Cut them into bite-sized pieces so they cook faster and more evenly.

- Add softer vegetables like tomatoes, mushrooms, and zucchini during the last 45 minutes of cooking time if you don't want them to be very soft.

- Buy roasts and other large cuts of meat that will fit in your slow cooker or trim them to fit. Trim extra fat from meat. This is not only healthier, but it will allow the meat to cook more evenly.

- Use cheaper cuts of meat. Not only do you save money, but these meats work better in the slow cooker. Cheaper cuts of meat have less fat, which makes them more suited to slow-cooker cooking. Moist, long cooking times result in very tender meats.

- Ground meat should usually be browned before adding it to the slow cooker. Larger pieces of meat can be browned before cooking, but this step isn't necessary. Browning will add color and flavor.

•	Remove the skin from poultry. It will end up flabby and rubbery anyway, and it contains the majority of the fat in poultry.

•	Seafood should usually be added during the last hour of cooking time, or it will overcook and have a rubbery texture.

•	Dairy products should usually be added during the last half hour of cooking time. They tend to break down if cooked too long.

•	Long-grain converted rice works best for long cooking times. If using rice, you should not reduce the amount of liquid when converting a recipe for the slow cooker.

- Pasta quickly overcooks in the slow cooker. Cook pasta separately until it is just starting to soften and then add it during the last half hour of cooking.

- You can thicken the juices by removing the lid and cooking on high for the last half hour of cooking time. If there is a lot of liquid to be thickened, dissolve a tablespoon or two of cornstarch in cold water and stir it in when you turn the heat to high.

- Slow cookers sometimes dilute flavors over a long period because of the amount of moisture generated. Taste and add more garlic powder, onion powder, pepper, or herbs and spices as needed near the end of cooking.

- At altitudes above 3,500 feet (1 km), you may need to add 30 minutes or more to the cooking time.

Slow Cooker Safety

There have been questions raised about the safety of cooking at low temperatures. It is true that if food is held at too low a temperature for too long, bacteria that would be a health concern could grow. However, used properly the slow cooker produces a safe cooking environment. Follow these tips to ensure that you don't have any problems.

- Keep food refrigerated before putting it in the slow cooker. Having food at room temperature provides an environment that is conducive to bacteria growth.

- Thaw frozen foods before placing them in the slow cooker to allow it to get to the proper operating temperature.

- To get the food up to temperature faster, heat the liquid before adding it to the cooker.

- If possible, cook on high for the first hour to get the food temperature up, and then reduce to low for the remainder of the time. Some newer cooker models can be programmed to do this automatically.

- Keep the lid on to help maintain the temperature. Resist the temptation to peek; it will be all right on its own.

- If your cooker has a "keep warm" setting, use that to maintain the food temperature once cooking is finished. If not, remove the food when the cooker is finished and refrigerate any leftovers promptly.

- To check that your cooker heats properly, fill it two-thirds full of water, turn it to low, cover, and let it cook for 8 hours without removing the lid. Remove the lid and check the temperature with a cooking thermometer. The water temperature should be at least 170 degrees Fahrenheit (77 degrees Celsius).

Converting Recipes for the Slow Cooker

Many regular recipes can be successfully converted to use the slow cooker. Some types of food flt the slow cooking method better than others. Because you generally need some liquid, foods like soups, stews, and roasts are usually good candidates. The following guidelines will help you in converting your favorite recipes to the slow cooker.

- Many slow cooker recipes recommend cooking for 8 to 10 hours on low, so this is usually a good starting point. Some recipes recommend using the high setting based on the food. For example, beef cuts will be better when cooked on low for 8 to 10 hours to get a more tender texture, while chicken can be cooked on high for 2^ to 3 hours.

- One hour of cooking on the high setting is approximately equal to 2 to 2^ hours on low.

- Reduce the amount of liquid used in most oven recipes when using the slow cooker since it retains moisture that usually evaporates when cooking in the oven. You will normally end up with more liquid at the end of the cooking time, not less. A general rule is to reduce liquids by half, unless rice or pasta is in the dish.

• Herbs and spices may need to be increased. Ground spices tend to lose some flavor during the long cooking. Add ground spices during the last hour of cooking to avoid this.

• Pasta, seafood, and milk do not hold up well during long cooking. Add these about 2 hours before the end when using the low setting or 1 hour on high. Evaporated milk can be added at the beginning of cooking.

• Dry beans can be soaked or cooked overnight on low in the slow cooker. Drain and combine with other ingredients. If your recipe includes tomatoes or other acidic ingredients, make sure the beans are tender before adding the acidic foods.

- Dense vegetables like potatoes, carrots, and other root vegetables should be cut no larger than 1 inch (2.5 cm) thick and placed in the bottom of the pot since they take longer to cook.

- If the conventional cooking time is 15 to 30 minutes, cooking time in a slower cooker on low should be about 4 to 6 hours.

- If the conventional cooking time is 30 to 60 minutes, cooking time in a slow cooker on low should be about 6 to 8 hours.

- If the conventional cooking time is 1 to 3 hours, cooking time in a slow cooker on low should be about 8 to 16 hours.

Slow Cooker Chickpea & Lentil Curry

Ingredients:

- 2 tablespoons olive oil

- 1 onion, chopped

- 2 cloves garlic, minced

- 1 teaspoon ground ginger

- 1 teaspoon ground cumin

- 1 teaspoon ground coriander

- 2 teaspoons ground turmeric

- 1 teaspoon chili powder

- 1 (14.5-ounce) can diced tomatoes

- 1 cup dried chickpeas, soaked overnight

- 1 cup dried lentils

- 4 cups vegetable broth

- 2 tablespoons tomato paste

- Salt and pepper, to taste

- 2 tablespoons chopped fresh cilantro

Instructions:

1. Heat the oil in a large skillet over medium-high heat. Add the onion and garlic and cook until softened, about 5 minutes.

2. Add the ginger, cumin, coriander, turmeric, and chili powder and cook for another minute.

3. Transfer the mixture to a slow cooker. Add the diced tomatoes, chickpeas, lentils, vegetable broth, and tomato paste.

4. Cover and cook on low for 8-10 hours or on high for 4-6 hours, until the chickpeas and lentils are tender.

5. Season with salt and pepper, to taste. Serve over cooked rice or quinoa and garnish with fresh cilantro.

Prep Time: 10 minutes

Cook Time: 8-10 hours

Yield: 6 servings

Nutritional Value: Calories: 300; Total Fat: 8 g; Saturated Fat: 1 g; Cholesterol: 0 mg; Sodium: 590 mg; Carbohydrates: 37 g; Fiber: 15 g; Sugar: 6 g; Protein: 17 g.

write 10 creative and powerful heart-healthy slow cooker recipes with instructions, prep time, yield and nutrional value

1. Curried Vegetable Stew:

Prep Time: 10 minutes

Cook Time: 6-8 hours

Yield: 6 servings

Nutritional Value: Calories: 230, Fat: 5g, Carbs: 41g, Protein: 8g

Ingredients:

-1 onion, chopped

-2 cloves garlic, minced

-1 tablespoon curry powder

-2 carrots, chopped

-2 potatoes, chopped

-1 cup green beans, trimmed and cut into 1-inch

pieces

-1 cup frozen corn kernels

-1 can (14.5 ounces) diced tomatoes

-1 can (14.5 ounces) low-sodium vegetable broth

-1 can (15 ounces) chickpeas, drained and rinsed

-Salt and pepper, to taste

-2 tablespoons fresh parsley, chopped (optional)

Instructions:

1. Place onion, garlic, and curry powder into a slow cooker and stir to combine.

2. Add carrots, potatoes, green beans, corn, tomatoes, broth, and chickpeas. Stir to combine.

3. Cover and cook on low for 6-8 hours.

4. Season with salt and pepper, to taste.

5. Sprinkle with fresh parsley before serving, if desired.

2. Vegetarian Chili:

Prep Time: 10 minutes

Cook Time: 8-10 hours

Yield: 8 servings

Nutritional Value: Calories: 246, Fat: 5g, Carbs: 39g, Protein: 11g

Ingredients:

-1 onion, diced

-2 cloves garlic, minced

-1 red bell pepper, diced

-1 green bell pepper, diced

-1 jalapeño pepper, seeded and minced

-1 can (14.5 ounces) diced tomatoes

-1 can (15.5 ounces) black beans, drained and rinsed

-1 can (15.5 ounces) kidney beans, drained and rinsed

-1 can (14.5 ounces) low-sodium vegetable broth

-1 tablespoon chili powder

-1 teaspoon ground cumin

-Salt and pepper, to taste

-2 tablespoons fresh cilantro, chopped (optional)

Instructions:

1. Place onion, garlic, bell peppers, jalapeño, tomatoes, beans, broth, chili powder, and cumin into a slow cooker and stir to combine.

2. Cover and cook on low for 8-10 hours.

3. Season with salt and pepper, to taste.

4. Sprinkle with fresh cilantro before serving, if desired.

3. Lentil Soup:

Prep Time: 10 minutes

Cook Time: 6-8 hours

Yield: 6 servings

Nutritional Value: Calories: 167, Fat: 1g, Carbs: 29g, Protein: 9g

Ingredients:

-1 onion, diced

-2 cloves garlic, minced

-2 carrots, diced

-2 stalks celery, diced

-1 cup dried green lentils, rinsed

-1 can (14.5 ounces) diced tomatoes

-4 cups low-sodium vegetable broth

-1 teaspoon dried thyme

-Salt and pepper, to taste

-2 tablespoons fresh parsley, chopped (optional)

Instructions:

1. Place onion, garlic, carrots, celery, lentils, tomatoes, broth, and thyme into a slow cooker and stir to combine.

2. Cover and cook on low for 6-8 hours.

3. Season with salt and pepper, to taste.

4. Sprinkle with fresh parsley before serving, if desired.

4. Hearty Minestrone Soup:

Prep Time: 10 minutes

Cook Time: 6-8 hours

Yield: 6 servings

Nutritional Value: Calories: 189, Fat: 2g, Carbs: 33g, Protein: 10g

Ingredients:

-1 onion, diced

-2 cloves garlic, minced

-2 carrots, diced

-2 stalks celery, diced

-1 zucchini, diced

-1 can (14.5 ounces) diced tomatoes

-1 can (15.5 ounces) chickpeas, drained and rinsed

-4 cups low-sodium vegetable broth

-1 teaspoon dried oregano

-1 teaspoon dried basil

-Salt and pepper, to taste

-2 tablespoons fresh parsley, chopped (optional)

Instructions:

1. Place onion, garlic, carrots, celery, zucchini, tomatoes, chickpeas, broth, oregano, and basil into a slow cooker and stir to combine.

2. Cover and cook on low for 6-8 hours.

3. Season with salt and pepper, to taste.

4. Sprinkle with fresh parsley before serving, if desired.

5. Mushroom Barley Soup:

Prep Time: 10 minutes

Cook Time: 6-8 hours

Yield: 6 servings

Nutritional Value: Calories: 228, Fat: 3g, Carbs: 43g, Protein: 10g

Ingredients:

-1 onion, diced

-2 cloves garlic, minced

-2 carrots, diced

-2 stalks celery, diced

-1 cup mushrooms, sliced

-1/2 cup pearled barley

-1 can (14.5 ounces) diced tomatoes

-4 cups low-sodium vegetable broth

-1 teaspoon dried thyme

-Salt and pepper, to taste

-2 tablespoons fresh parsley, chopped (optional)

Instructions:

1. Place onion, garlic, carrots, celery, mushrooms, barley, tomatoes, broth, and thyme into a slow cooker and stir to combine.

2. Cover and cook on low for 6-8 hours.

3. Season with salt and pepper, to taste.

4. Sprinkle with fresh parsley before serving, if desired.

6. Chickpea Curry:

Prep Time: 10 minutes

Cook Time: 6-8 hours

Yield: 6 servings

Nutritional Value: Calories: 255, Fat: 6g, Carbs: 40g, Protein: 11g

Ingredients:

-1 onion, diced

-2 cloves garlic, minced

-1 tablespoon curry powder

-1 tablespoon ginger, grated

-2 carrots, diced

-1 can (14.5 ounces) diced tomatoes

-1 can (15.5 ounces) chickpeas, drained and

rinsed

-1 cup coconut milk

-Salt and pepper, to taste

-2 tablespoons fresh cilantro, chopped (optional)

Instructions:

1. Place onion, garlic, curry powder, ginger, carrots, tomatoes, chickpeas, and coconut milk into a slow cooker and stir to combine.

2. Cover and cook on low for 6-8 hours.

3. Season with salt and pepper, to taste.

4. Sprinkle with fresh cilantro before serving, if desired.

7. Mexican Quinoa:

Prep Time: 10 minutes

Cook Time: 6-8 hours

Yield: 6 servings

Nutritional Value: Calories: 238, Fat: 5g, Carbs: 38g, Protein: 9g

Ingredients:

-1 onion, diced

-2 cloves garlic, minced

-1 red bell pepper, diced

-1 can (14.5 ounces) diced tomatoes

-1 cup quinoa, rinsed

-1 can (15.5 ounces) black beans, drained and rinsed

-1 can (14.5 ounces) low-sodium vegetable broth

-1 teaspoon chili powder

-1 teaspoon ground cumin

-Salt and pepper, to taste

-2 tablespoons fresh cilantro, chopped (optional)

Instructions:

1. Place onion, garlic, bell pepper, tomatoes, quinoa, beans, broth, chili powder, and cumin into a slow cooker and stir to combine.

2. Cover and cook on low for 6-8 hours.

3. Season with salt and pepper, to taste.

4. Sprinkle with fresh cilantro before serving, if desired.

8. Split Pea Soup:

Prep Time: 10 minutes

Cook Time: 6-8 hours

Yield: 6 servings

Nutritional Value: Calories: 190, Fat: 1g, Carbs: 33g, Protein: 11g

Ingredients:

-1 onion, diced

-2 cloves garlic, minced

-2 carrots, diced

-2 stalks celery, diced

-1 cup dried split peas, rinsed

-1 can (14.5 ounces) diced tomatoes

-4 cups low-sodium vegetable broth

-1 teaspoon dried thyme

-Salt and pepper, to taste

-2 tablespoons fresh parsley, chopped (optional)

Instructions:

1. Place onion, garlic, carrots, celery, split peas, tomatoes, broth, and thyme into a slow cooker and stir to combine.

2. Cover and cook on low for 6-8 hours.

3. Season with salt and pepper, to taste.

4. Sprinkle with fresh parsley before serving, if desired.

9. Butternut Squash Soup:

Prep Time: 10 minutes

Cook Time: 6-8 hours

Yield: 6 servings

Nutritional Value: Calories: 150, Fat: 4g, Carbs: 26g, Protein: 3g

Ingredients:

-1 onion, diced

-2 cloves garlic, minced

-2 carrots, diced

-2 stalks celery, diced

-1 butternut squash, peeled, seeded, and cubed

-1 can (14.5 ounces) diced tomatoes

-4 cups low-sodium vegetable broth

-1 teaspoon dried thyme

-Salt and pepper, to taste

-2 tablespoons fresh parsley, chopped (optional)

Instructions:

1. Place onion, garlic, carrots, celery, butternut squash, tomatoes, broth, and thyme into a slow cooker and stir to combine.

2. Cover and cook on low for 6-8 hours.

3. Season with salt and pepper, to taste.

4. Sprinkle with fresh parsley before serving, if desired.

10. Sweet Potato Soup:

Prep Time: 10 minutes

Cook Time: 6-8 hours

Yield: 6 servings

Nutritional Value: Calories: 175, Fat: 5g, Carbs: 32g, Protein: 4g

Ingredients:

-1 onion, diced

-2 cloves garlic, minced

-2 carrots, diced

-2 stalks celery, diced

-3 sweet potatoes, peeled and cubed

-1 can (14.5 ounces) diced tomatoes

-4 cups low-sodium vegetable broth

-1 teaspoon dried thyme

-Salt and pepper, to taste

-2 tablespoons fresh parsley, chopped (optional)

Instructions:

1. Place onion, garlic, carrots, celery, sweet potatoes, tomatoes, broth, and thyme into a slow cooker and stir to combine.

2. Cover and cook on low for 6-8 hours.

3. Season with salt and pepper, to taste.

4. Sprinkle with fresh parsley before serving, if desired.

Tender and Tasty Low-Fat Beef Main Dishes Easy and Lean

1 Sweet Potato and Lentil Stew:

Ingredients: 2 sweet potatoes, peeled and diced; 1 cup of dried lentils; 1 onion, diced; 2 cloves of garlic, minced; 2 cups of low-sodium beef broth; ½ teaspoon of smoked paprika; 2 tablespoons of olive oil; Salt and pepper to taste.

Instructions: Heat the olive oil in the bottom of a slow cooker. Add the onion, garlic, sweet potatoes and lentils and stir to combine. Pour in the beef broth and add the smoked paprika. Gently stir to make sure all the ingredients are evenly distributed. Cover the slow cooker and cook on low heat for 8-10 hours, or until the lentils and sweet potatoes are fully cooked. Season with salt and pepper to taste.

Prep Time: 10 minutes

Yield: 4 servings

Nutritional Value: Calories: 230; Total Fat: 5 g; Saturated Fat: 1 g; Cholesterol: 0 mg; Sodium: 120 mg; Carbohydrates: 34 g; Fiber: 11 g; Protein: 12 g.

2. Slow Cooker Pot Roast:

Ingredients: 2.5 pounds of lean beef chuck roast; 2 cups of low-sodium beef broth; 1 onion, diced; 2 cloves of garlic, minced; 2 carrots, peeled and diced; 2 stalks of celery, diced; 1 teaspoon of

Worcestershire sauce; 2 tablespoons of olive oil; Salt and pepper to taste.

Instructions: Heat the olive oil in the bottom of a slow cooker. Add the onion, garlic, carrots, celery, and beef chuck roast and stir to combine. Pour in the beef broth and Worcestershire sauce. Gently stir to make sure all the ingredients are evenly distributed. Cover the slow cooker and cook on low heat for 8-10 hours, or until the beef is fully cooked and tender. Season with salt and pepper to taste.

Prep Time: 10 minutes

Yield: 8 servings

Nutritional Value: Calories: 284; Total Fat: 14 g; Saturated Fat: 4 g; Cholesterol: 72 mg; Sodium:

120 mg; Carbohydrates: 3 g; Fiber: 1 g; Protein: 33 g.

3. Beef and Mushroom Stew:

Ingredients: 2 pounds of lean beef chuck, cubed; 8 ounces of mushrooms, sliced; 2 cloves of garlic, minced; 2 cups of low-sodium beef broth; 2 tablespoons of tomato paste; 2 tablespoons of olive oil; Salt and pepper to taste.

Instructions: Heat the olive oil in the bottom of a slow cooker. Add the beef cubes and mushrooms and stir to combine. Pour in the beef broth and tomato paste. Gently stir to make sure all the ingredients are evenly distributed. Cover the slow cooker and cook on low heat for 8-10 hours, or until the beef cubes are fully cooked and tender. Season with salt and pepper to taste.

Prep Time: 10 minutes

Yield: 6 servings

Nutritional Value: Calories: 234; Total Fat: 11 g; Saturated Fat: 4 g; Cholesterol: 68 mg; Sodium: 120 mg; Carbohydrates: 4 g; Fiber: 0 g; Protein: 28 g.

4. Beef and Kale Stew:

Ingredients: 2 pounds of lean beef chuck, cubed; 2 bunches of kale, stems removed and chopped; 2 cloves of garlic, minced; 2 cups of low-sodium beef broth; 2 tablespoons of tomato paste; 2 tablespoons of olive oil; Salt and pepper to taste.

Instructions: Heat the olive oil in the bottom of a slow cooker. Add the beef cubes and kale and stir to combine. Pour in the beef broth and tomato paste. Gently stir to make sure all the ingredients are evenly distributed. Cover the slow cooker and cook on low heat for 8-10 hours, or until the beef cubes are fully cooked and tender. Season with salt and pepper to taste.

Prep Time: 10 minutes

Yield: 8 servings

Nutritional Value: Calories: 234; Total Fat: 11 g; Saturated Fat: 4 g; Cholesterol: 68 mg; Sodium: 120 mg; Carbohydrates: 6 g; Fiber: 2 g; Protein: 28 g.

5. Hearty Beef and Vegetable Stew:

Ingredients: 2 pounds of lean beef chuck, cubed; 2 cups of diced potatoes; 1 cup of diced carrots; 1 cup of diced celery; 2 cloves of garlic, minced; 2 cups of low-sodium beef broth; 2 tablespoons of tomato paste; 2 tablespoons of olive oil; Salt and pepper to taste.

Instructions: Heat the olive oil in the bottom of a slow cooker. Add the beef cubes, potatoes, carrots, celery and garlic and stir to combine. Pour in the beef broth and tomato paste. Gently stir to make sure all the ingredients are evenly distributed. Cover the slow cooker and cook on low heat for 8-10 hours, or until the beef cubes are fully cooked and tender. Season with salt and pepper to taste.

Prep Time: 10 minutes

Yield: 8 servings

Nutritional Value: Calories: 220; Total Fat: 9 g; Saturated Fat: 3 g; Cholesterol: 65 mg; Sodium: 120 mg; Carbohydrates: 16 g; Fiber: 2 g; Protein: 22 g.

6. Slow Cooker Beef Chili:

Ingredients: 2 pounds of lean ground beef; 1 onion, diced; 2 cloves of garlic, minced; 2 cups of low-sodium beef broth; 1 can of diced tomatoes; 2 tablespoons of chili powder; 2 tablespoons of olive oil; Salt and pepper to taste.

Instructions: Heat the olive oil in the bottom of a slow cooker. Add the ground beef, onion, garlic, beef broth and diced tomatoes. Gently stir to make sure all the ingredients are evenly distributed. Cover the slow cooker and cook on low heat for 8-10 hours, or until the beef cubes are fully cooked and tender. Stir in the chili powder, season with salt and pepper to taste.

Prep Time: 10 minutes

Yield: 8 servings

Nutritional Value: Calories: 252; Total Fat: 15 g; Saturated Fat: 4 g; Cholesterol: 72 mg; Sodium: 120 mg; Carbohydrates: 8 g; Fiber: 2 g; Protein: 25 g.

7. Slow Cooker Stuffed Peppers:

Ingredients: 4 large bell peppers, halved and seeded; 2 cups of cooked brown rice; 2 pounds of lean ground beef; 1 onion, diced; 2 cloves of garlic, minced; 2 cups of low-sodium beef broth; 1 can of diced tomatoes; 2 tablespoons of olive oil; Salt and pepper to taste.

Instructions: Heat the olive oil in the bottom of a slow cooker. Add the ground beef, onion, garlic, beef broth and diced tomatoes. Gently stir to make sure all the ingredients are evenly distributed. Place the bell pepper halves in the slow cooker, fill each one with cooked brown rice. Cover the slow cooker and cook on low heat for 8-10 hours, or until the beef cubes are fully cooked and tender. Season with salt and pepper to taste.

Prep Time: 10 minutes

Yield: 8 servings

Nutritional Value: Calories: 252; Total Fat: 14 g; Saturated Fat: 4 g; Cholesterol: 72 mg; Sodium: 120 mg; Carbohydrates: 17 g; Fiber: 3 g; Protein: 19 g.

8. Beef and Barley Stew:

Ingredients: 2 pounds of lean beef chuck, cubed; 1 cup of pearl barley; 2 cloves of garlic, minced; 2 cups of low-sodium beef broth; 2 tablespoons of tomato paste; 2 tablespoons of olive oil; Salt and pepper to taste.

Instructions: Heat the olive oil in the bottom of a slow cooker. Add the beef cubes and pearl barley and stir to combine. Pour in the beef broth and tomato paste. Gently stir to make sure all the ingredients are evenly distributed. Cover the slow cooker and cook on low heat for 8-10 hours, or until the beef cubes are fully cooked and tender. Season with salt and pepper to taste.

Prep Time: 10 minutes

Yield: 8 servings

Nutritional Value: Calories: 234; Total Fat: 11 g; Saturated Fat: 4 g; Cholesterol: 68 mg; Sodium: 120 mg; Carbohydrates: 16 g; Fiber: 3 g; Protein: 28 g.

9. Slow Cooker Beef Stroganoff:

Ingredients: 2 pounds of lean beef chuck, cubed; 2 cups of sliced mushrooms; 2 cloves of garlic, minced; 2 cups of low-sodium beef broth; 2 tablespoons of tomato paste; 1 cup of Greek yogurt; 2 tablespoons of olive oil; Salt and pepper to taste.

Instructions: Heat the olive oil in the bottom of a slow cooker. Add the beef cubes, mushrooms and garlic and stir to combine. Pour in the beef broth and tomato paste. Gently stir to make sure all the ingredients are evenly distributed. Cover the slow cooker and cook on low heat for 8-10 hours, or until the beef cubes are fully cooked and tender. Stir in the Greek yogurt and season with salt and pepper to taste.

Prep Time: 10 minutes

Yield: 8 servings

Nutritional Value: Calories: 252; Total Fat: 14 g; Saturated Fat: 4 g; Cholesterol: 72 mg; Sodium: 120 mg; Carbohydrates: 6 g; Fiber: 1 g; Protein: 28 g.

10. Slow Cooker Beef and Butternut Squash Stew:

Ingredients: 2 pounds of lean beef chuck, cubed; 2 cups of diced butternut squash; 2 cloves of garlic, minced; 2 cups of low-sodium beef broth; 2 tablespoons of tomato paste; 2 tablespoons of olive oil; Salt and pepper to taste.

Instructions: Heat the olive oil in the bottom of a slow cooker. Add the beef cubes, butternut squash and garlic and stir to combine. Pour in the beef broth and tomato paste. Gently stir to make sure all the ingredients are evenly distributed. Cover the slow cooker and cook on low heat for 8-10 hours, or until the beef cubes are fully cooked and tender. Season with salt and pepper to taste.

Prep Time: 10 minutes

Yield: 8 servings

Nutritional Value: Calories: 220; Total Fat: 9 g; Saturated Fat: 3 g; Cholesterol: 65 mg; Sodium: 120 mg; Carbohydrates: 13 g; Fiber: 2 g; Protein: 22 g.